MEAL PREP C

CW00518507

Recipe book for beginners to prepare easy and healthy meals for weight loss and to prepare a weekly program of ready meals

Table of Contents

INTRODUCTION **8**

How to Meal Prep? 10
Mint Shrimp 13
Baked Salmon and Asparagus in Garlic Lemon Olive Sauce 15
Caramelized Tuna 17
Fig Crusted Cod 18
Celery Cilantro Tuna Stew 21
Roasted Cauliflower Broccoli Salmon Bowl 22
Coconut Lime Scallops 25
Baked Lemon Cod 26
Pan-Fried Apricot Salmon Bites 27
Bass with Crispy Sweet Potato Crust 28
Fish and Leek Sauté 30
Cilantro Lime Shrimp Quinoa Bowl 31
Ahi Tuna and Spicy Salmon Poke Bowl 33
Lemon Roasted Salmon with Sweet Potatoes & Broccolini 35
Cranberry Balsamic Salmon 38
Paprika Salmon and Green Beans 40
Braised Salmon in Creamy Mushroom Sauce 43
Caramelized Asian BBQ Salmon 45
Sun-Dried Tomato Lemon Baked Salmon & Asparagus 48
Parmesan and Herb Crusted Fish 50

POULTRY **52**

Curry Chicken Salad 54
Rolled Pesto Chicken 55
Chicken Divan Casserole 58
Bacon and Onion Chicken Breasts 60
Pizza Chicken 62
Jerk Chicken 65
Italian Herb Chicken 67
Buffalo Bleu Cheese Chicken Burgers 68
Thai Peanut Chicken and "Rice" 70
Chicken Tandoori 72
Baked Garlic Chicken 75
Chicken Makhani 76
Bacon-Roasted Chicken 79
Prosciutto-Wrapped Mushroom Chicken 80
Indian Chicken Thighs 82
Rosemary-Roasted Turkey 84
Spinach and Cheese Turkey Pinwheels 86

MOZZARELLA-STUFFED TURKEY MEATBALLS.. 88
TURKEY BACON CHEESEBURGER MEATLOAF.. 90
BAKED CHICKEN 92
ORANGE CHICKEN AND BROCCOLI STIR-FRY.. 94
MEDITERRANEAN LEMON CHICKEN AND POTATOES 96
TANDOORI CHICKEN 97
GRILLED CHICKEN SALAD 99
GROUND TURKEY MINI MEATLOAVES 101
TURKEY AND BROWN RICE STUFFED PEPPERS 103
GRILLED TEQUILA CHICKEN WITH PEPPERS.. 105
ORANGE-ROSEMARY ROASTED CHICKEN... 107
HONEY CRUSTED CHICKEN 108

The information in the following pages is broadly considered a truthful and accurate account of facts and as such, any inattention, use, or misuse of the information in question by the reader will render any resulting actions solely under their purview. There are no scenarios in which the publisher or the original author of this work can be in any fashion deemed liable for any hardship or damages that may befall them after undertaking information described herein.

Additionally, the information in the following pages is intended only for informational purposes and should thus be thought of as universal. As befitting its nature, it is presented without assurance regarding its prolonged validity or interim quality. Trademarks that are mentioned are done without written consent and can in no way be considered an endorsement from the trademark holder.

Introduction

Why is this Meal Prep Cookbook release so important? Because at MEAL PREP, we believe in the power of preparing today's foods with the assurance that you'll always have healthy options to get the body and mind ready for tomorrow. This cookbook is full of easy recipes that will save you money and help you achieve your fitness goals.

In recent years, Meal Prep has become an emerging trend as people realize the benefits of spending time preparing meals in advance. Convenience, cost-effectiveness, and time-saving are the main factors contributing to the growing popularity of meal prep. If you are a busy working professional, meal prep will help you cut down on the money and time you spend on buying take-outs from the office cafeteria. It will also help you stay away from junk food and better control your caloric intake. Preparing a few portions of your favorite meals can help you save money and feel energetic enough to make it through the long and busy work schedule and daily responsibilities.

The most significant advantage of prepping your own meals is the chance to personalize your meals. This factor makes prepping meals more enjoyable and exciting. Individuals used to buy prepared meals from their local grocery stores and take their meals to work. It cost money and took up most of their time only to have it eaten in front of them while they are sitting at their desks all day.

While the benefits of meal prep can be split into two main categories: financial and health, it saves lots of your finances in the long run by reaping the benefits of cheaper food. You will also enjoy healthier eating because you already chose what and how much to eat. Not to mention, meal prep is an excellent way to stay consistent with your goals and objectives. For anyone who wants to lose weight, for example, the key to long-term success is consistency. To succeed with weight loss, you must stay in control of your diet. If you are going about it the right way and planning ahead, you will lose weight much easier than you ever thought possible.

It also allows you to eat healthy throughout the week without worrying about finding time to shop or cook. This meal prep cookbook includes a wide range of recipes so that you can use this book for multiple purposes. You can use these recipes for meal prepping, as well as making them from scratch for your family and friends.

How to Meal Prep?

There are different ways on how you can meal prep if you're a beginner in this journey. Some of them are the following:

Make-Ahead Meals

Prepare for the week ahead and freeze the meals that you plan to cook every week. This kind of meal preparation is easy and saves time in the summer. Using freezer containers is a great way to preserve food for future use. The frozen meals taste great and have fewer ingredients. You will also save your wallet on fresh groceries.

Batch Cooking

This meal prep method involves preparing multiple recipes at a time and cooking them all together. It is an excellent way to prepare several meals fast. This method's advantage is that it is economical since you can prepare large portions of food in one go.

Individually Portioned Meals

Prepare food individually and make sure they will be ready fast. This method is perfect for a week filled with celebrations. You can prepare each meal individually in the evening and enjoy the benefits of eating right out of the containers.

Ready-To-Cook Ingredients

If you're a busy person who does not have much time to cook in the morning, shopping for ready-to-cook ingredients will do. Buying and preparing fresh ingredients ahead of time will help you save time in the busy mornings. But make sure to eat fresh meals. As soon as the ingredients are bought, they will also spoil if not eaten straight away. Therefore, you need to plan your meals ahead of time to make sure you will use them before they get stale.

Now that you know the basics and advantages of meal prepping, it's time to get down to the most awaited 500 meal prep recipes with the 30-day meal plan by the end of it. We hope you'll enjoy the wide range of meals but make sure to make them in your own way. If you are a vegan, don't add meat to your recipes. If you are a vegetarian, add some meat to the recipe. Most importantly, don't fear to play around with your recipes! Happy meal prepping.

Mint Shrimp

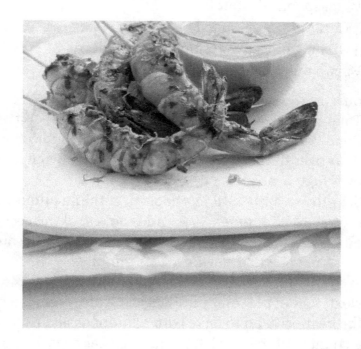

Preparation time: 15 minutes
Cooking time: 10 minutes
Servings: 3
Ingredients:

- ¼ tablespoon Fish Sauce
- 1 1/2 tablespoons coconut oil divided
- 3/4-pound shrimp
- ¼ teaspoon Salt
- ¼ teaspoon coconut flour
- 4 Garlic cloves chopped
- 3 Green Onions whites only, thinly sliced
- ¼ cup mint leaves packed

Directions:

1. Take the fish sauce in a small bowl and then set it aside. Pour 1 tablespoon of the coconut oil, salt, and coconut flour over the shrimp and then toss. Warm your wok over high heat.
2. Sear the shrimp until just cooked, within 2 minutes, then remove, and set aside. Add the rest of the coconut oil in the pan and the garlic, onion, plus the fish sauce mixture and stir-fry within a few minutes.
3. Toss the shrimp back in and stir-fry within few minutes. Next, fold in the mint until it's just wilted, remove from the heat—season to taste with additional salt. Store an airtight container or heavy-duty freezer bags for up to 3 months in the freezer and 3-4 days in the fridge.

Nutrition:
Calories 178
Fat 7.2g
Carbohydrate 3.5g
Protein 21g

Baked Salmon and Asparagus in Garlic Lemon Olive Sauce

Preparation time: 15 minutes
Cooking time: 20 minutes
Servings: 3
Ingredients:

- 3 fillets salmon
- ½ lb. asparagus, ends trimmed
- salt
- ½ teaspoon Italian seasoning, thyme
- 42 garlic cloves, minced
- ½ lemon, thinly sliced
- 1/8 cup olive, drained
- 2 tablespoons butter

Directions:

1. Warm oven to 400 F. Prepares s 3 separate foil pieces; large enough to cover each fish fillet when folded.
2. Put equal portions of asparagus in the center of each foil; season asparagus with salt. Put each fish fillet on top of asparagus.
3. Flavor each fillet with a pinch of Italian herbal seasoning, salt, and sprinkle minced garlic over each fillet and asparagus.
4. Top each salmon fillet with a thin lemon slice; sprinkle 1 tablespoon of olive over each fillet. Put each fillet with 1 tablespoon butter on top, thinly sliced.
5. Wrap the foil ends over the salmon to enclose it but do not wrap too tightly - leave some space.
6. Put foil-wrapped fish fillets on a baking sheet. Bake within 20 minutes at 400 F until the salmon is cooked through and flaky.

7. Store an airtight container or heavy-duty freezer bags for up to 3 days in the fridge.

Nutrition:
Calories 298
Fat 17.6g
Carbohydrate 13.6g
Protein 23.4g

Caramelized Tuna

Preparation time: 15 minutes
Cooking time: 20 minutes
Servings: 3
Ingredients:

- ¼ cup of coconut sugar
- 1 tablespoon of sea salt
- 4 tuna Fillets
- 2 tablespoons Olive oil

Directions:

1. Combine your coconut sugar and sea salt in a small bowl. Put your olive oil in a medium skillet and heat over medium heat.
2. Take your tuna fillets and apply your spice rub evenly all over when your oil is hot, place your fillet in the pan cooking within two minutes on each side.
3. Store an airtight container or heavy-duty freezer bags up to 3-4 days in the fridge, 2-3 months in the freezer.

Nutrition:
Calories 181
Fat 15.1g
Carbohydrate 0.9g

Fig Crusted Cod

Preparation time: 15 minutes
Cooking time: 22 minutes
Servings: 3
Ingredients:

- 1-pound cod – cut into portions
- 3 dried figs- chopped
- 1 date – pitted
- 1/2 cup water
- 1/8 teaspoon cinnamon powder
- 1/4 teaspoon pink Himalayan salt
- 1/2 tablespoon garlic powder
- 1/4 cup orange juice, squeezed

Directions:

1. Warm oven to 350F. Prepare a roasting pan with parchment paper and place cod (skin side down) on paper. Set aside.
2. Make fig topping, lace all other fixings in a saucepan and bring to a low boil. Simmer within 5 minutes, or until most of the liquid is cooked off. Move to a food processor and process to a smooth consistency.
3. Spread the fig topping on the fish. Bake within 18-22 – depending on the thickness of cod pieces and how well done you like your cod. Let cod rest on stovetop or counter within 3-4 minutes to finish cooking.
4. Serve with roasted veggies and a simple salad for a complete meal. Store an airtight container or heavy-duty freezer bags up to 3-4 days in the fridge, 2-3 months in the freezer.

Nutrition:
Calories 98

Fat 0.6g
Carbohydrate 9.9g
Protein 13.5g

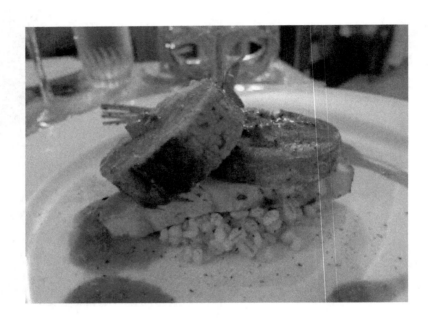

Celery Cilantro Tuna Stew

Preparation time: 15 minutes
Cooking time: 20 minutes
Servings: 3
Ingredients:

- 1 ½ cups water
- 1 ½ tuna filets, diced
- ¾ yellow squash, diced
- 1 ½ button mushrooms, diced
- ¾ cups chopped celery
- 1/4 cup chopped cilantro
- salt to taste

Directions:

1. Place all the vegetables with the water into a pot and simmer for 15 minutes. Add the diced tuna and simmer for another 5 minutes.
2. Store an airtight container or heavy-duty freezer bags up to 3-4 days in the fridge, 2-3 months in the freezer.

Nutrition:
Calories 169
Fat 11.4g
Carbohydrate 5g
Protein 12.3g

Roasted Cauliflower Broccoli Salmon Bowl

Preparation time: 15 minutes
Cooking time: 20 minutes
Servings: 3
Ingredients:
- ¾ head of cauliflower, broken into small florets
- ¾ head of broccoli, broken into small florets
- Coconut oil to cook with
- ¼ lemon
- Salt to taste
- 1 ½ (5-oz) cans of salmon
- ¼ cup fresh basil, finely chopped

Directions:
1. Warm oven to 400 F. Put the cauliflower plus broccoli florets on a baking tray and drizzle coconut oil over them.
2. Flavor with salt plus juice from 1/4 lemon over the vegetables. Massage the mixture into your vegetables using your hands and put it over the baking tray.
3. Place into the oven and cook within or 20 minutes.
4. Let the vegetables cool within a few minutes, then place them into a large bowl and toss with the chopped basil, 1 tablespoon coconut oil, juice from 1/4 lemon, and extra salt to taste.
5. To serve, put the roasted vegetables into a small bowl with salmon. Store an airtight container or heavy-duty freezer bags up to 3-4 days in the fridge, 2-3 months in the freezer.

Nutrition:
Calories 43

Fat 1.4g
Carbohydrate 3.2g
Protein 5.1g

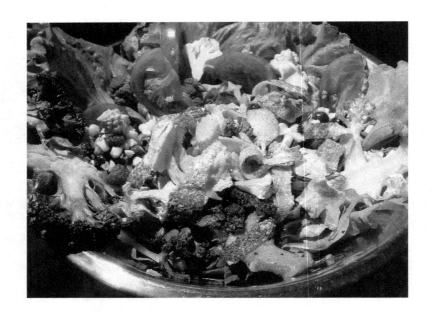

Coconut Lime Scallops

Preparation time: 15 minutes
Cooking time: 5 minutes
Servings: 3
Ingredients:

- 1 1/2 tablespoons of coconut flour
- 1/4 cup of coconut flakes
- 6 oz of scallops
- coconut oil, for frying
- salt
- lime wedges, to serve

Directions:

1. Mix the coconut flour plus coconut in a bowl. Add the scallops and press the coconut into the scallops well.
2. Heat oil for deep-frying the shrimp. Place a scallop in the oil. Fry within 1-2 minutes. Remove, then place on a tray or plate lined with a paper towel.
3. Serve warm, flavor with salt and a generous squeeze of lime. Store an airtight container or heavy-duty freezer bags up to 3-4 days in the fridge, 2-3 months in the freezer.

Nutrition:
Calories 115
Fat 4.5g
Carbohydrate 5.4g
Protein 13.2g

Baked Lemon Cod

Preparation time: 15 minutes
Cooking time: 20 minutes
Servings: 3
Ingredients:

- ½ Lemons, sliced thinly
- 1 1/2 lbs. Filets of cod, fresh or frozen
- ¾ tablespoons of coconut oil
- Salt
- basil sprigs, to garnish
- Beetroot salad, to serve

Directions:

1. Warm oven to 350°F. Split the lemon slices in half. Put one-half of the lemons on a sheet of foil. Put the cod over the lemons, then cover using the second half. Put olive oil over the fillets.
2. Fold the foil over the fillets, seal—Bake in the oven within 20 minutes. Season the cod with salt and serve garnished with basil alongside a fresh green beetroot salad.
3. Store an airtight container or heavy-duty freezer bags up to 3-4 days in the fridge, 2-3 months in the freezer.

Nutrition:
Calories 79
Fat 3.9g
Carbohydrate 1.4g
Protein 10.2g

Pan-Fried Apricot Salmon Bites

Preparation time: 15 minutes
Cooking time: 5 minutes
Servings: 3
Ingredients:

- 3 apricots, sliced in half and stones removed
- ¾ cans salmon, flaked
- ¾ tablespoons thyme leaves, diced
- ¾ tablespoons olive oil
- Sea salt
- Coconut oil
- 3 blackberries, sliced in half

Directions:

1. Put the coconut oil into your frying pan and pan-fry the apricot halves cut-face down, so they're slightly browned. Alternatively, you can grill the apricot halves instead.
2. In a bowl, mix the salmon, thyme leaves, olive oil, and sea salt to taste. Use a spoon to pile mounds of the salmon mixture on top of the apricot halves.
3. Top each salmon apricot bite with half a blackberry. Store an airtight container or heavy-duty freezer bags up to 3-4 days in the fridge, 2-3 months in the freezer.

Nutrition:
Calories 110
Fat 7g
Carbohydrate 3.7g
Protein 9.1g

Bass with Crispy Sweet Potato Crust

Preparation time: 15 minutes
Cooking time: 10 minutes
Servings: 3
Ingredients:
- 1-1/4 tablespoons olive oil
- ¾ medium sweet potato, peeled and grated)
- 3 bass fillets, about 6 ounces each
- salt, to taste

Directions:
1. Heat-up oil over medium-high in a large, non-stick skillet. Add eight "nests" of the grated sweet potato, roughly in the shape of the fillets'
2. Put the fillets over the nests, then let it cook until the sweet potatoes' edges are browned.
3. Flip each piece of fish with its crust using a large spatula. Continue cooking until the fish is cooked through.
4. Sprinkle with salt and serve. Store an airtight container or heavy-duty freezer bags up to 3-4 days in the fridge, 2-3 months in the freezer.

Nutrition:
Calories 185
Fat 11.6g
Carbohydrate 4.7g
Protein 16g

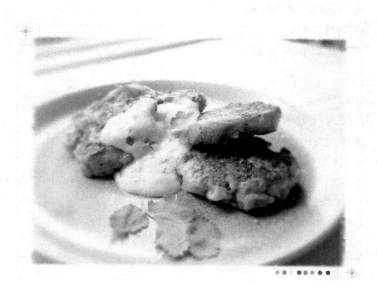

Fish and Leek Sauté

Preparation time: 15 minutes
Cooking time: 10 minutes
Servings: 3
Ingredients:
- 1-1/2 fish fillets diced
- ¾ leeks, chopped
- ¼ teaspoon grated ginger
- ¾ tablespoons coconut aminos
- Salt to taste
- ¾ tablespoons olive oil

Directions:
1. Add the olive oil into a skillet and sauté the chopped leek. When the leeks soften, add in the diced fish, grated ginger, coconut aminos, and salt to taste.
2. Sauté until the fish isn't translucent anymore and is cooked. Serve. Store an airtight container or heavy-duty freezer bags up to 3-4 days in the fridge, 2-3 months in the freezer.

Nutrition:
Calories 154
Fat 9.2g
Carbohydrate 11.8g
Protein 7g

Cilantro Lime Shrimp Quinoa Bowl

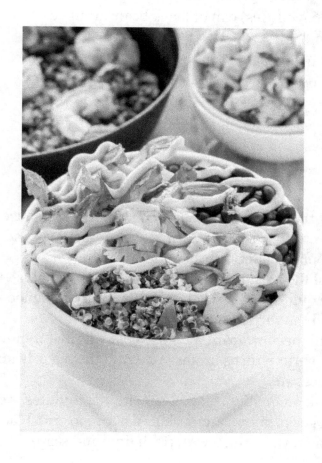

Preparation time: 15 minutes
Cooking time: 15 minutes
Servings: 2 to 4
Ingredients:

- 1 pound of shrimp peeled and deveined
- 2 cups of quinoa cooked
- 1 (16.5 ounces) can of black beans drained
- 1 lime juice
- ½ cup of cilantro chopped
- 1 avocado sliced
- 1 teaspoon of low-sodium soy sauce
- 1 teaspoon of lemon pepper seasoning
- 1 teaspoon of barbeque seasoning
- Salt and pepper to taste

Directions:

1. Put the shrimp in a Ziploc bag. Put the soy sauce plus juice from the lime. Sprinkle the seasonings and chopped cilantro throughout.
2. Seal the bag and refrigerate within 45 minutes—Cook the quinoa. Remove the shrimp from the Ziploc and load the shrimp into a grill pan.
3. Grill the shrimp on medium heat within 4 minutes until the shrimp turns bright pink. Add the black beans to a saucepan.
4. Cook on medium-high heat within 4 minutes. Add the cooked shrimp, quinoa, sliced avocado, and black beans to a bowl. Garnish with fresh lime and serve.

Nutrition:
Calories: 537
Carbs: 70g
Fat: 16g
Protein: 30g

Ahi Tuna and Spicy Salmon Poke Bowl

Preparation time: 15 minutes
Cooking time: 45 minutes
Servings: 2 to 4
Ingredients:

- 1 ½ cups of raw short-grain brown rice
- 2 tbsp. of seasoned rice vinegar
- ½ lb. of sushi-grade yellowfin tuna
- 1 tbsp. of thinly sliced scallion (white and green parts)
- 1 tsp. of very thinly sliced shallot
- 2 tsp. of reduced-sodium tamari
- 1 tsp. of toasted sesame oil
- Pinch of chili flakes
- ½ lb. of sushi-grade salmon
- 2 tsp. of mayonnaise
- Sriracha to taste -- start with ¼ teaspoon
- ¼ tsp. of reduced-sodium tamari
- 1 tsp. of finely minced shallot
- 1 tbsp. of sliced scallions
- Sliced avocado
- Prepared seaweed salad
- Fish roe
- Shelled edamame
- Toasted nori
- Furikake or gomasio
- Toasted sesame oil (with or without chili)

Directions:

1. Put the rice plus 3 cups of water into a medium pot and allow to boil. Cover then adjust the heat to maintain a gentle simmer.

2. Cook within 45 minutes, until water is absorbed and rice is tender. Let the rice rest, covered, within 10 minutes, then stir in vinegar.

3. For the tuna poke, slice tuna into bite-sized cubes, maybe ½ inch dice. Put cubes in a small mixing bowl and add scallion, shallot, tamari, sesame oil, and chili flakes.

4. Toss gently and set it aside. For the salmon poke, slice salmon into cubes and put it in a small mixing bowl.

5. Stir the mayonnaise, sriracha, and tamari in another small bowl. Spoon sauce over your salmon and toss to coat.

6. Stir in shallot and scallion and set it aside. Assemble the bowls by placing some rice in the bottom of your serving bowl.

7. Arrange portions of tuna, salmon, plus whatever additional fixings you like avocado, shelled edamame, a bit of salmon roe, plus a sprinkle of gomasio, freshly ground black pepper, and chili toasted sesame oil. Serve immediately and Enjoy!

Nutrition:
Calories: 790
Carbs: 103g
Fat: 41g
Protein: 32g

Lemon Roasted Salmon with Sweet Potatoes & Broccolini

Preparation time: 15 minutes
Cooking time: 30 minutes
Servings: 5
Ingredients:

- 2 medium sweet potatoes, cubed
- Sea salt + fresh black pepper
- ½ tsp. of cumin powder
- 2 tbsp. of olive oil
- 4 cups of broccolini (or broccoli florets)
- 12 oz. of wild-caught salmon filets
- 1 tbsp. of butter
- 2 tbsp. of lemon juice
- ¼ tsp. of garlic powder
- 1/8 tsp. of red pepper flakes and fresh thyme (optional)

Directions:

1. Preheat the oven to 425°F and arrange the chopped sweet potatoes on your sheet pan plus the broccolini on another sheet pan, put both with olive oil.
2. Top the sweet potatoes with salt, pepper, plus cumin, toss. Toss the broccolini with the salt plus pepper.
3. Bake the sweet potatoes for about 15 minutes, set the broccolini aside.
4. Prepare the salmon by mixing the butter, lemon juice, garlic powder, pepper flakes, thyme, salt, and pepper in a small bowl.
5. Heat in the microwave for 15 seconds more. Prepare a small baking sheet with foil, oiled with cooking spray.

6. Put the salmon filets on top. Put the prepared lemon sauce. Remove the sweet potatoes from cooking, then toss.
7. Put back in the oven with the broccolini plus salmon for about 15 minutes. Check on the salmon plus broccolini around the 8-minute mark.
8. Split the veggies and salmon into containers and allow to cool slightly before refrigerating and serve!

Nutrition:
Calories: 105
Carbs: 21g
Fat: 3g
Protein: 3g

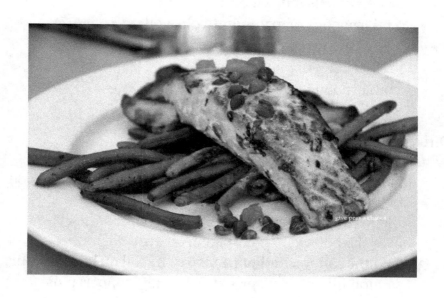

Cranberry Balsamic Salmon

Preparation time: 5 minutes
Cooking time: 20 minutes
Servings: 1 to 3
Ingredients:

- 2 salmon fillets
- 1 cup of fresh or frozen (thawed) cranberries + 2 tbsp more (divided)
- ¼ cup of balsamic vinegar
- 2 tablespoons of extra virgin olive oil
- 2 tablespoons of orange juice
- 1 tablespoon of maple syrup
- 1 tablespoon of rosemary
- Salt & pepper to taste

Directions:

1. Preheat oven to 3500F. Put 1 cup of cranberries, balsamic, orange juice, maple syrup in a blender or food processor.
2. Blend on high for about 2 minutes. Spread the glaze over the bottom of your pan in an even layer.
3. Add the salmon and put 1 tbsp of the oil on each of your salmon fillets, then sprinkle with salt, pepper, plus rosemary.
4. Put the extra two tablespoons of cranberries around your salmon in the sauce place it in the oven to bake at 350 F within 18 minutes.
5. Turn the oven off and turn the broiler on high. Boil for about 3 minutes until glaze is thick and the fish is flaky. Remove from the oven, serve, and enjoy!

Nutrition:
Calories: 257

Carbs: 14g
Fat: 26g
Protein: 23g

Paprika Salmon and Green Beans

Preparation time: 10 minutes
Cooking Time: 15 minutes
Servings: 1 to 3
Ingredients:

- 3 Salmon steaks room temperature (5 oz.)
- ¼ cup of canola oil or more
- 2 tsp of minced garlic
- ½ tbsp. of onion powder
- 1 tbsp. of smoked paprika
- ½ tsp. of cayenne pepper optional
- 3 tbsp. of fresh herbs thyme, parsley, basil
- ½ tsp. of bouillon powder
- 1 lb. of green beans and carrots or any vegetables.
- Salt and pepper to taste

Directions:

1. Prepare a rack in the middle of your oven and warm the oven to 400°F. Line a baking sheet with foil and cooking spray and set it aside.
2. Mix canola oil, minced garlic, fresh herbs, smoked paprika, onion powder, and cayenne pepper in a small pan set over medium-low heat.
3. Stir for about 2 minutes. Let this mixture rest for a little bit within 5 minutes. Put the salmon in a large bowl; salt then tosses with garlic paprika spice mixture.
4. Put on your prepared baking sheet, repeat the same process with the vegetable next to the salmon, depending on your baking sheet. Allow the salmon to bake for about 18 minutes, serve or store.

Nutrition:
Calories: 300

Carbs: 15g
Fat: 24g
Protein: 9g

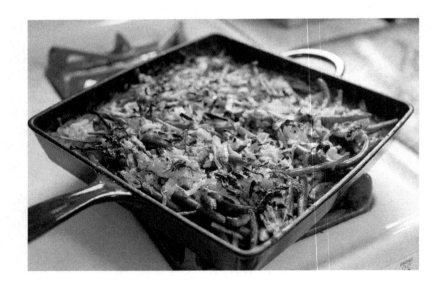

Braised Salmon in Creamy Mushroom Sauce

Preparation time: 10 minutes
Cooking time: 30 minutes
Servings: 2 to 4
Ingredients:
- 5 tablespoons of ghee
- 4 salmon fillets (skinless)
- Salt & pepper
- Paprika
- 1 onion (sliced)
- 2 garlic cloves (finely minced)
- 1 red jalapeno pepper (diced)
- 4 oz. of shitake mushrooms (sliced)
- 1 tablespoon of coconut aminos
- 1 cup of coconut milk
- ¼ cup of seafood stock
- 1 cup of baby spinach leaves
- 1 teaspoon of cayenne pepper

Directions:
1. Heat-up 2 tablespoons of ghee in a large cast-iron pan over medium-high heat and flavor each salmon fillet with salt, pepper, and paprika.
2. Then, sear salmon for approximately 3 minutes on each side. Remove salmon from the pan and set it aside. Put another 2 tablespoons of ghee in the pan and sauté onions, garlic, and jalapeno peppers.
3. Flavor with a pinch of salt plus pepper and sauté until onions are tender, then add mushrooms and coconut aminos.

4. Stir in the extra teaspoon of ghee and continue to cook (stirring frequently) until mushrooms are tender.
5. Now stir in seafood, coconut milk, spinach, and cayenne pepper. Nestle salmon into the sauce and simmer for about 7 minutes until sauce thickens a bit.
6. Turn the oven to broil, then move the skillet to the oven. Broil for 5 minutes to add some color to the fish. Serve with roasted veggies, potatoes, noodles, or a salad.

Nutrition:
Calories: 582
Carbs: 14g
Fat: 38g
Protein: 38g

Caramelized Asian BBQ Salmon

Preparation time: 5 minutes
Cooking time: 9 minutes
Servings: 2 to 4
Ingredients:

- 4 skinless salmon fillets (6oz. each)
- 1 tbsp. of toasted sesame oil, divided

Marinade:

- 2 tbsp. of Asian sweet chili sauce
- 3 tbsp. of ketchup
- 3 tbsp. of quality hoisin sauce
- 2 tbsp. of cider vinegar
- 2 tbsp. of brown sugar
- 2 tbsp. of soy sauce
- 2 tsp. of freshly grated ginger
- ½ tsp. of garlic powder
- ½ tsp. of sriracha

Directions:

1. Whisk all of the marinade/glaze fixings plus 2 teaspoon sesame oil. Put 1/3 cup of marinade in a freezer bag with salmon.
2. Fridge the rest separately and marinate salmon for one hour or overnight when ready to cook; let salmon sit at room temperature within 10 minutes.
3. Split reserved glaze in half; heat-up 1 teaspoon sesame oil in a 12-inch non-stick skillet over medium-high heat. Put the salmon and adjust to medium heat and sear until the side is browned for about 4 minutes.
4. Flip salmon over and spoon half the rest of the glaze over salmon. Cook for an additional 7 minutes depending on thickness and desired doneness.

5. Spoon the desired amount of remaining glaze over individual servings and season with freshly cracked salt and pepper. Serve immediately and Enjoy!

Nutrition:
Calories: 278
Carbs: 2g
Fat: 17g
Protein: 30g

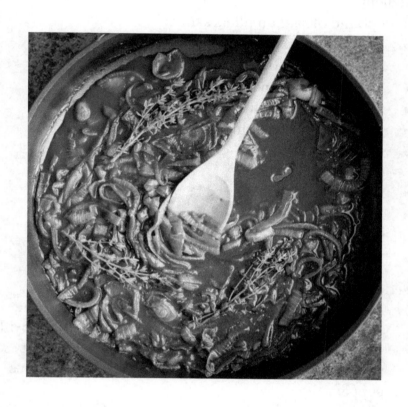

Sun-Dried Tomato Lemon Baked Salmon & Asparagus

Preparation time: 5 minutes
Cooking time: 20 minutes
Servings: 1 to 3
Ingredients:

- 1 pound of salmon fillets skin on
- 10 ounces of asparagus
- Zest from 1 lemon
- Juice from ½ lemon
- 2 tablespoons of olive oil
- 3 tablespoons dry white wine
- 3 ounces of diced sun-dried tomatoes in olive oil just tomatoes
- 1 teaspoon of dry crushed basil
- 4 large garlic cloves
- Salt
- Fresh cracked black pepper

Directions:

1. Preheat the oven to 4250F and line a rimmed baking sheet with parchment paper. Massage salmon skin with some oil, then put salmon fillets on your parchment paper, skin down. Flavor salmon with a little salt plus pepper.
2. Slice the white edges of the asparagus off, then slice the stalks in half. Put asparagus on the baking sheet in 1 layer, around salmon.
3. Mix lemon zest, lemon juice, olive oil, wine, sun-dried tomatoes, pressed garlic, dry basil, salt, and pepper in a small bowl.

4. Whisk and spoon the sauce batter over salmon and asparagus. Bake within 20 minutes, depending on the thickness of salmon fillets.

Nutrition:
Calories: 291
Carbs: 4g
Fat: 20g
Protein: 24g

Parmesan and Herb Crusted Fish

Preparation time: 7 minutes
Cooking time: 10 minutes
Servings: 1 to 3
Ingredients:

- 8 oz. of fillet of white fish (or tilapia)
- ¼ cup of shredded parmesan cheese
- ½ tbsp. of butter
- ½ tsp. of oregano
- ½ tsp. of thyme
- ½ tsp. of rosemary

Directions:

1. Put fish skin side down on a baking sheet. Toss the parmesan, oregano, thyme, and rosemary in a small bowl.
2. Dissolve the butter in the microwave. Brush your butter on the upright side of the fish in another small bowl.
3. Sprinkle with the parmesan, then herb mixture. Set your broiler to high heat; put fish on a broiler rack under the flame.
4. Let it broil for about 10 minutes or until golden brown, and the fish has reached an internal temperature of at least 145 degrees. Serve immediately and Enjoy!

Nutrition:
Calories: 160
Carbs: 9g
Fat: 6g
Protein: 26g

Poultry

Feta Cheese Turkey Burgers

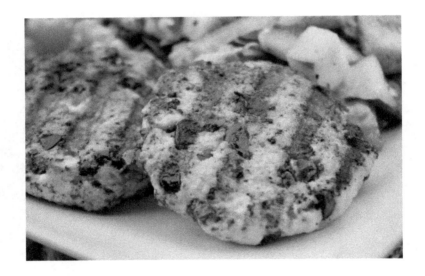

Preparation time: 15 minutes
Cooking time: 10 minutes
Servings: 5
Ingredients:

- 11/2 pounds ground turkey
- 11/2 cups crumbled feta cheese
- 1 clove garlic, minced
- 1/4 cup chicken bone broth
- 1/2 cup Kalamata olives, pitted & minced
- 2 teaspoons Greek seasoning
- 1/2 teaspoon freshly ground black pepper
- 2 tablespoons avocado oil

Directions:

1. Combine all fixings, except oil, in a medium bowl. Use your hands to mix until incorporated. Form into six patties.
2. Heat-up oil in a medium skillet over medium heat. Transfer patties to the hot pan and cook for 5 minutes on each side.
3. Remove, then allow to cool slightly. Transfer each burger to a separate airtight container and store in the refrigerator until ready to eat, up to one week.

Nutrition:
Calories: 318
Fat: 21 g
Protein: 27 g
Carbohydrates: 5 g

Curry Chicken Salad

Preparation time: 15 minutes
Cooking time: 0 minutes
Servings: 6
Ingredients:

- 11/2 pounds chicken breasts, boneless & skinless, cooked and diced
- 2 medium stalks celery, finely chopped
- 1/2 medium white onion, peeled and minced
- 1/2 cup toasted walnuts
- 1/4 teaspoon freshly ground black pepper
- 1/2 teaspoon curry powder
- 3/4 cup coconut oil mayonnaise

Directions:

1. Combine all fixings in a medium bowl and stir until evenly incorporated.
2. Split into six equal portions and move each portion to a separate airtight container. Put in the refrigerator until ready to eat, up to one week.

Nutrition:
Calories: 206
Fat: 9 g
Protein: 26 g
Carbohydrates: 3 g

Rolled Pesto Chicken

Preparation time: 15 minutes
Cooking time: 45 minutes
Servings: 6
Ingredients:

- 2 cups fresh basil
- 3 cloves garlic
- 1 tablespoon pine nuts
- 1/4 cup whole milk ricotta cheese
- 1/4 cup grated Parmesan cheese
- 21/2 tablespoons olive oil
- 1/2 teaspoon sea salt
- 1/4 teaspoon freshly ground black pepper
- 6 (4-ounce) boneless, skinless chicken breasts
- 6 slices provolone cheese

Directions:

1. Preheat oven to 350°F. Mix basil, garlic, plus pine nuts in a food processor and process until chopped.
2. Add ricotta cheese and process until incorporated. Put parmesan cheese, olive oil, salt, plus pepper and process until smooth.
3. Butterfly each chicken breast and pound to 1/4" thickness. Spread 3 tablespoons of prepared pesto onto each flattened chicken breast and place 1 slice of cheese on top of the pesto.
4. Roll chicken breast tightly and secure in place with toothpicks. Transfer each chicken breast to a 9" × 13" baking dish.
5. Bake 45 minutes or until chicken is cooked through. Allow to cool and transfer each chicken breast to a separate airtight container. Put in the refrigerator for up to one week.

Nutrition:
Calories: 338
Fat: 20 g
Protein: 35 g
Carbohydrates: 3 g

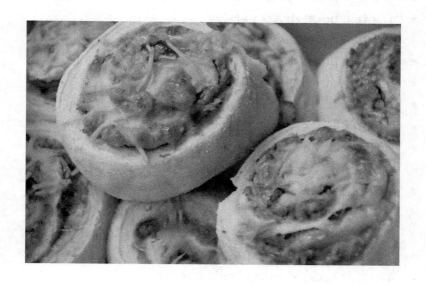

Chicken Divan Casserole

Preparation time: 15 minutes
Cooking time: 1 hour & 10 minutes
Servings: 6
Ingredients:

- 3 tablespoons grass-fed butter
- 1 small yellow onion, peeled and diced
- 2 teaspoons minced garlic
- 1/2 teaspoon garlic salt
- 1/4 teaspoon dried parsley
- 1/4 teaspoon sea salt
- 1/4 teaspoon freshly ground black pepper
- 2 cups cauliflower rice
- 1 cup of chicken bone broth
- 1 cup heavy cream
- 1 teaspoon lemon juice
- 1/2 cup mayonnaise
- 11/2 pounds chicken breasts, boneless & skinless, cooked and shredded
- 4 cups broccoli florets, steamed and chopped
- 1 cup shredded Cheddar cheese
- 1 cup shredded mozzarella cheese

Directions:

1. Preheat oven to 350°F. Dissolve the butter in a medium saucepan over medium heat. Put onion plus garlic and cook until softened, about 6 minutes. Stir in garlic salt, parsley, sea salt, and pepper.
2. Add cauliflower rice and chicken bone broth and cook until most broth has been absorbed into the cauliflower, about 10 minutes.

3. Mix in heavy cream plus lemon juice and reduce heat to low. Simmer 10 minutes. Remove from heat and stir in mayonnaise.
4. Spread cooked chicken in the bottom of a 9" × 13" pan and pour half of the sauce on top. Stir to combine and then spread out again. Layer chopped broccoli on top and pour remaining sauce over broccoli.
5. Sprinkle cheeses on top—cover and bake for 30 minutes. Remove cover, then bake within 10 more minutes or until cheese starts to brown on edges.
6. Allow cooling, then slice into six equal portions. Move each portion to a different airtight container and store in the refrigerator until ready to eat, up to one week.

Nutrition:
Calories: 642
Fat: 50 g
Protein: 38 g
Carbohydrates: 9 g

Bacon and Onion Chicken Breasts

Preparation time: 15 minutes
Cooking time: 30 minutes
Servings: 6
Ingredients:
- 1 pound no-sugar-added bacon
- 1 large yellow onion, peeled and sliced
- 1/4 cup granulated erythritol
- 2 teaspoons coconut aminos
- 1/4 teaspoon sea salt
- 1/2 teaspoon lemon pepper seasoning
- 6 (4-ounce) boneless, skinless chicken breasts
- 2 tablespoons avocado oil
- 1 cup shredded Monterey jack cheese

Directions:
1. Preheat oven to 350°F. Cook the bacon in your large skillet on medium-high heat. Transfer to a paper towel-lined plate and reserve bacon grease.
2. Add onion, erythritol, and coconut aminos to the hot pan and cook until onions are caramelized about 10 minutes.
3. Chop bacon and stir into onion mixture. Sprinkle salt and lemon pepper over chicken breasts and add avocado oil to a clean medium skillet over medium heat.
4. Put the chicken in the pan, cook 7 minutes, flip over, and cook another 8 minutes.
5. Top each of your chicken breasts with equal parts of the onion and bacon mixture. Put cheese on top of each breast, then cover skillet until cheese melts, about 3 minutes.

6. Remove chicken, then allow to cool. Transfer each breast to an airtight container and store in the refrigerator until ready to eat, up to one week.

Nutrition:
Calories: 585
Fat: 44 g
Protein: 40 g
Carbohydrates: 11 g

Pizza Chicken

Preparation time: 15 minutes
Cooking time: 30 minutes
Servings: 6
Ingredients:

- 1 cup crushed pork rinds
- 1 teaspoon Italian seasoning
- 3/4 cup grated Parmesan cheese
- 1 teaspoon of sea salt
- 1 teaspoon freshly ground black pepper
- 1 cup almond flour
- 1 teaspoon granulated garlic
- 1 teaspoon granulated onion
- 3 large eggs
- 3 tablespoons lemon juice
- 6 (4-ounce) boneless, skinless chicken breasts
- 11/2 cups no-sugar-added pizza sauce
- 18 slices pepperoni
- 11/2 cups shredded mozzarella cheese

Directions:

1. Preheat oven to 400°F. Combine pork rinds, Italian seasoning, Parmesan cheese, salt, and pepper in a medium bowl.
2. Combine almond flour, granulated garlic, and granulated onion in a separate medium bowl. Whisk together eggs and lemon juice in a third medium bowl.
3. Dip each chicken breast in egg batter, then cover with almond flour mixture. Dip in the egg mixture a second time and then coat with pork rinds.
4. Place coated chicken breasts in a 9" × 13" baking dish and bake 20 minutes.

5. Spoon equal amounts of pizza sauce onto each chicken breast. Put 3 pieces of pepperoni on top of pizza sauce, and sprinkle mozzarella cheese on top.
6. Bake 10 more minutes. Remove from oven and allow to cool. Transfer each chicken breast to a separate airtight container and store in the refrigerator until ready to eat, up to one week.

Nutrition:
Calories: 437
Fat: 18 g
Protein: 42 g
Carbohydrates: 8 g

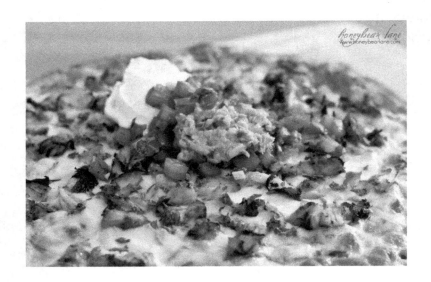

Jerk Chicken

Preparation time: 15 minutes
Cooking time: 15 minutes
Servings: 6
Ingredients:

- 2 teaspoons finely minced white onion
- 1/4 cup granulated erythritol
- 1/4 cup coconut aminos
- 1/4 cup red wine vinegar
- 1 teaspoon dried thyme
- 2 teaspoons sesame oil
- 4 cloves garlic, minced
- 3/4 teaspoon ground allspice
- 1 habanero pepper, sliced
- 1 1/2 pounds chicken thighs, boneless, skinless, cut into strips

Directions:

1. Combine onion, erythritol, coconut aminos, red wine vinegar, thyme, sesame oil, garlic, allspice, and habanero in a food processor and process until smooth.
2. Move 3/4 of the batter to a sealable bag and add chicken strips. Massage to coat and refrigerate for 1 hour.
3. Turn your oven on broil. While the oven is preheating, transfer chicken to a baking sheet. Broil 7 minutes, flip the chicken over and broil an additional 8 minutes.
4. Remove chicken from oven and pour reserved jerk sauce on top. Allow to cool, then transfer equal portions to six separate airtight containers. Put in the refrigerator until ready to eat, up to one week.

Nutrition:

Calories: 155
Fat: 6 g
Protein: 22 g
Carbohydrates: 9g

Italian Herb Chicken

Preparation time: 15 minutes
Cooking time: 40 minutes
Servings: 6
Ingredients:
- 6 (4-ounce) boneless, skinless chicken breasts
- 3 tablespoons Italian seasoning
- 1 teaspoon of sea salt
- 3/4 teaspoon crushed red pepper
- 6 cloves garlic, minced
- 3 Roma tomatoes, sliced thinly
- 1/2 cup crumbled feta cheese

Directions:
1. Preheat oven to 350°F. Oiled a 9" × 13" baking dish with cooking spray. Place chicken breasts in the prepared baking dish and sprinkle Italian seasoning, salt, and red pepper over them.
2. Top chicken with minced garlic and sliced tomato and cover. Bake 25 minutes. Remove cover, sprinkle feta on top of each chicken breast, and bake another 15 minutes or until chicken is cooked through.
3. Allow to cool and then transfer each chicken breast to a separate airtight container. Put in the refrigerator until ready to eat, up to one week.

Nutrition:
Calories: 178
Fat: 6 g
Protein: 27g
Carbohydrates: 3g

Buffalo Bleu Cheese Chicken Burgers

Preparation time: 15 minutes
Cooking time: 20 minutes
Servings: 6
Ingredients:

- 11/2 pounds ground chicken
- 11/2 cups almond meal
- 3/4 cup crumbled blue cheese
- 1 large egg
- 2 tablespoons dried minced onion
- 1/2 cup Frank's Red Hot sauce

Directions:

1. Combine all fixings in a medium bowl and mix with your hands until incorporated. Refrigerate for 1 hour. Preheat oven to 350°F. Line a baking sheet with parchment paper.
2. Form mixture into six patties and transfer to the prepared baking sheet. Bake 20 minutes, or until chicken reaches an internal temperature of 165°F, flipping once during cooking.
3. Allow to cool and transfer each patty to a separate airtight container. Put in the refrigerator until ready to eat, up to one week.

Nutrition:
Calories: 436
Fat: 24 g
Protein: 26 g
Carbohydrates: 6 g

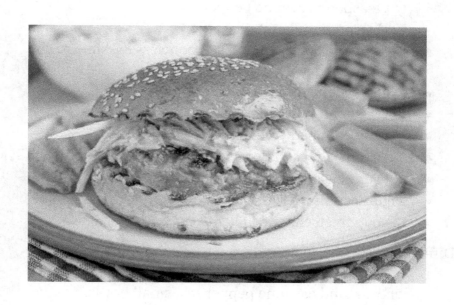

Thai Peanut Chicken and "Rice"

Preparation time: 15 minutes
Cooking time: 15 minutes
Servings: 6
Ingredients:

- 6 tablespoons coconut aminos
- 4 tablespoons no-sugar-added creamy peanut butter
- 4 teaspoons white wine vinegar
- 1/4 teaspoon cayenne pepper
- 3 tablespoons peanut oil
- 1 1/2 pounds chicken breasts, boneless & skinless, cut into thin strips
- 2 tablespoons minced garlic
- 1 tablespoon minced fresh ginger
- 1/2 cup chopped green onion
- 2 1/2 cups broccoli florets
- 1/3 cup roasted peanuts
- 2 cups cauliflower rice
- 1/2 cup fresh chopped cilantro

Directions:

1. Combine coconut aminos, peanut butter, white wine vinegar, and cayenne pepper in a small bowl and stir until mixed. Set aside.
2. Heat-up peanut oil in a medium skillet or wok over high heat. Add chicken, garlic, ginger, and cook until the chicken starts to brown, about 5 minutes.
3. Reduce to medium heat and put green onion, broccoli, peanuts, and peanut butter sauce. Cook 5 minutes, stirring constantly.

4. Add cauliflower rice and cook another 4 minutes, or until cauliflower and broccoli are tender, and chicken is cooked through. Stir in cilantro and remove from heat.
5. Split into six equal portions and move each portion to a separate airtight container. Put in the refrigerator until ready to eat, up to one week.

Nutrition:
Calories: 342
Fat: 20 g
Protein: 31 g
Carbohydrates: 10 g

Chicken Tandoori

Preparation time: 15 minutes
Cooking time: 25 minutes
Servings: 6
Ingredients:

- 11/4 cups plain Greek yogurt
- 11/2 teaspoons sea salt
- 1 teaspoon freshly ground black pepper
- 1/2 teaspoon ground cloves
- 1/2 teaspoon ground ginger
- 3 teaspoons paprika
- 2 teaspoons ground cumin
- 2 teaspoons ground coriander
- 2 teaspoons ground cinnamon
- 4 cloves garlic, minced
- 11/2 pounds boneless, skinless chicken thighs

Directions:

1. Combine yogurt, spices, and garlic in a small bowl and mix well. Transfer to a sealable bag and add chicken.
2. Squeeze excess air, seal tightly, and massage marinade and chicken together. Refrigerate overnight (or at least 8 hours).
3. Preheat oven to 350°F. Set a wire cake rack inside a rimmed baking sheet. Remove chicken from bag and wipe off most of the yogurt marinade, leaving a thin layer on chicken.
4. Arrange chicken on top of the wire rack. Bake 25 minutes, turn oven to broil, and bake 5 more minutes or until chicken is cooked through and crispy on the outside.
5. Remove from oven and allow to cool. Split into six equal portions and move each portion to a separate airtight

container. Put in the refrigerator until ready to eat, up to one week.

Nutrition:
Calories: 181
Fat: 6 g
Protein: 24 g
Carbohydrates: 5 g

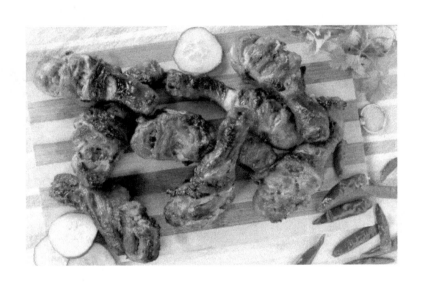

Baked Garlic Chicken

Preparation time: 15 minutes
Cooking time: 48 minutes
Servings: 6
Ingredients:
- 1/2 cup grass-fed butter
- 3 tablespoons coconut aminos
- 3 tablespoons minced garlic
- 1/4 teaspoon freshly ground black pepper
- 1 tablespoon dried rosemary
- 6 (4-ounce) boneless chicken thighs, skin on

Directions:
1. Preheat oven to 375°F. Combine butter, coconut aminos, garlic, pepper, and rosemary in a small saucepan over low heat. Cook until butter is melted, within 3 minutes, stirring occasionally.
2. Place chicken in a medium baking pan and pour butter mixture on top. Bake 45 minutes, flipping once during cooking, or until chicken is cooked through. Allow cooling.
3. Transfer each chicken thigh to a separate airtight container and store in the refrigerator until ready to eat, up to one week.

Nutrition:
Calories: 279
Fat: 20 g
Protein: 22 g
Carbohydrates: 1 g

Chicken Makhani

Preparation time: 15 minutes
Cooking time: 32 minutes
Servings: 6
Ingredients:

- 2 tablespoons butter-flavored coconut oil, divided
- 1 medium shallot, minced
- 1/2 medium white onion, peeled and diced
- 2 tablespoons grass-fed butter
- 2 teaspoons lemon juice
- 1 tablespoon minced garlic
- 1 teaspoon minced fresh ginger
- 2 teaspoons garam masala, divided
- 1 teaspoon chili powder
- 1 teaspoon ground cumin
- 1 teaspoon ground coriander
- 1 bay leaf
- 1 cup tomato sauce
- 1 cup heavy cream
- 1/4 cup plain Greek yogurt
- 1/4 teaspoon cayenne pepper, divided
- 1/4 teaspoon sea salt
- 1/4 teaspoon freshly ground black pepper
- 11/2 pounds chicken breasts, boneless & skinless, cubed
- 1/4 cup finely ground cashews

Directions:

1. Heat-up 1 tablespoon coconut oil in a large saucepan over medium-high heat. Add shallot and onion and cook until softened, about 5 minutes.
2. Stir in butter, lemon juice, garlic, ginger, 1 teaspoon garam masala, chili powder, cumin, coriander, and bay

leaf. Cook 1 minute, then add tomato sauce, cooking another 3 minutes while stirring constantly.

3. Reduce heat to low and stir in cream, yogurt, 1/8 teaspoon cayenne pepper, sea salt, and black pepper. Simmer 10 minutes, stirring frequently. Remove from heat and set aside.

4. Heat remaining coconut oil in a medium skillet over medium heat. Sprinkle 1 teaspoon garam masala and 1/8 teaspoon cayenne pepper on chicken cubes and add them to the hot pan—Cook within 8 minutes, or until chicken is cooked through.

5. Stir tomato sauce into chicken. Add cashews and stir again. Adjust heat to low and simmer 8 minutes, or until sauce thickens.

6. Remove from heat and allow to cool. Split into six equal portions, then move each portion to a separate airtight container. Put in the refrigerator until ready to eat, up to one week.

Nutrition:
Calories: 408
Fat: 29 g
Protein: 28 g
Carbohydrates: 7.5 g

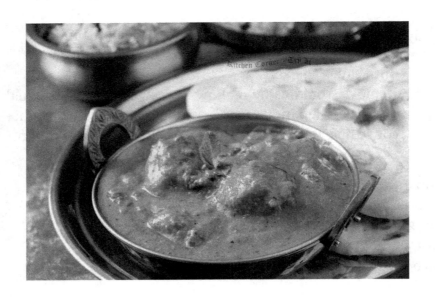

Bacon-Roasted Chicken

Preparation time: 15 minutes
Cooking time: 43 minutes
Servings: 6
Ingredients:

- 1 teaspoon of sea salt
- 1/2 teaspoon freshly ground black pepper
- 11/2 pounds boneless, skinless chicken thighs
- 12 slices no-sugar-added bacon
- 1 medium yellow onion, peeled & roughly chopped

Directions:

1. Preheat oven to 400°F. Sprinkle salt plus pepper all over chicken thighs. Wrap each thigh in bacon, covering as much of the chicken as possible. Secure in place with toothpicks.
2. Move the chicken to a 9" × 13" baking dish and sprinkle onions on top. Bake 40 minutes, turning once during cooking.
3. Switch oven to broil and bake again within 3 minutes on each side, or until bacon is crispy and chicken is cooked through.
4. Remove, then allow to cool slightly. Split into six equal portions and move each portion to a separate airtight container. Put in the refrigerator until ready to eat, up to one week.

Nutrition:
Calories: 376
Fat: 26 g
Protein: 29 g
Carbohydrates: 2.5 g

Prosciutto-Wrapped Mushroom Chicken

Preparation time: 15 minutes
Cooking time: 60 minutes
Servings: 6
Ingredients:

- 2 tablespoons grass-fed butter
- 1 cup sliced baby Bella mushrooms
- 1 medium yellow onion, peeled and chopped
- 1/2 teaspoon sea salt
- 1/4 teaspoon freshly ground black pepper
- 2 tablespoons minced garlic
- 6 (4-ounce) boneless, skinless chicken breasts
- 6 slices prosciutto, thinly sliced
- 1 cup full-fat sour cream
- 1/4 cup grated Asiago cheese

Directions:

1. Preheat oven to 350°F. Melt butter and drizzle into the bottom of a 9" × 13" baking dish. Spread mushrooms and onion out on the bottom of the buttered baking dish.
2. Combine sea salt, black pepper, and minced garlic in a small bowl and then spread over chicken. Cover each chicken breast with a cut of prosciutto and secure with a toothpick.
3. Bake 1 hour or until chicken is cooked through. Remove from oven and allow to cool—Transfer equal portions of chicken, mushrooms, and onion to each of six separate airtight containers.
4. Spoon pan juices into a small saucepan over low heat; stir in sour cream and Asiago cheese and continue

stirring until melted. Pour sauce over each portion of chicken.

5. Put in the refrigerator until ready to eat, up to one week.

Nutrition:
Calories: 386
Fat: 25 g
Protein: 33 g
Carbohydrates: 4.5 g

Indian Chicken Thighs

Preparation time: 15 minutes
Cooking time: 1 hour & 30 minutes
Servings: 6
Ingredients:

- 1 large yellow onion, peeled and diced
- 4 cloves garlic
- 1 (1") piece fresh ginger
- 2 tablespoons butter-flavored coconut oil
- 2 teaspoons ground cumin
- 1 teaspoon ground turmeric
- 1/2 teaspoon ground cardamom
- 1 teaspoon ground cinnamon
- 1/4 teaspoon ground cloves
- 1 teaspoon of sea salt
- 1 teaspoon freshly ground black pepper
- 6 (4-ounce) boneless, skinless chicken thighs
- 3 Roma tomatoes, diced and crushed

Directions:

1. Combine onion, garlic, plus ginger in a food processor and process until a paste form. Heat-up coconut oil in a medium skillet over medium heat.
2. Add onion mixture and sauté until softened, frequently stirring, for 5 minutes. Stir in spices and cook for another 2 minutes.
3. Place chicken thighs in skillet and spoon onion mixture over them until coated. Cook for 5 minutes and then pour in tomatoes and any juices released from crushing.
4. Reduce heat to low and simmer 45 minutes covered, and other 45 minutes uncovered.

5. Remove from heat and allow to cool. Transfer the chicken thighs to each of six separate airtight containers. Put in your ref for up to one week.

Nutrition:
Calories: 200
Fat: 9.5 g
Protein: 22 g
Carbohydrates: 5.5g

Rosemary-Roasted Turkey

Preparation time: 15 minutes
Cooking time: 2 hours & 30 minutes
Servings: 6
Ingredients:

- 1/2 cup olive oil
- 2 tablespoons minced garlic
- 2 tablespoons chopped fresh rosemary, plus 2 rosemary sprigs
- 1 tablespoon chopped fresh basil
- 1 tablespoon dried Italian seasoning
- 1 teaspoon of sea salt
- 1 teaspoon freshly ground black pepper
- 1 (6-pound) whole turkey
- 1 medium yellow onion, peeled and quartered
- 2 cups of chicken bone broth

Directions:

1. Preheat oven to 325°F. Combine olive oil, garlic, chopped rosemary, basil, Italian seasoning, salt, and pepper in a bowl and mix well.
2. Rub herbed oil batter all over the turkey, covering as much as you can. Place onion and rosemary sprigs in the turkey cavity.
3. Place turkey on a rack in a roast pan and add chicken broth to the pan's bottom. Roast within 2 1/2 hours or until internal temperature reaches 165°F. Allow to cool and remove meat from bones.
4. Split into six equal portions and move each portion to a separate airtight container. Put in the refrigerator until ready to eat, up to one week.

Nutrition:

Calories: 185
Fat: 18 g
Protein: 2 g
Carbohydrates: 4 g

Spinach and Cheese Turkey Pinwheels

Preparation time: 15 minutes
Cooking time: 60 minutes
Servings: 6
Ingredients:

- 11/2 pounds ground turkey
- 3/4 cup almond meal
- 1 large egg
- 11/4 teaspoons sea salt, divided
- 1/2 teaspoon freshly ground black pepper
- 1 package frozen chopped spinach, thawed & drained
- 3/4 cup shredded mozzarella cheese, divided
- 1/2 cup shredded provolone cheese
- 2 tablespoons grated Parmesan cheese
- 1 teaspoon Italian seasoning
- 1/4 teaspoon dried basil
- 1/4 teaspoon granulated garlic
- 1/4 cup no-sugar-added ketchup

Directions:

1. Preheat oven to 350°F. Prepare a baking sheet using parchment paper, then set aside.
2. Combine ground turkey, almond meal, egg, 1 teaspoon salt, and pepper in a medium bowl and mix with hands until incorporated.
3. Place turkey mixture on the prepared baking sheet and flatten it into a 10" × 14" rectangle.
4. Combine spinach, 1/2 cup mozzarella cheese, provolone cheese, Parmesan cheese, and remaining spices in a separate medium bowl. Stir to mix.
5. Spread spinach mixture over turkey, leaving 1/2" of space around the edges. Pick up one short edge of the parchment

paper and roll into a pinwheel, peeling back the parchment paper as you go. Pinch seam closed.

6. Place a wire rack in the baking sheet and place turkey pinwheel, seam side down, onto the rack. Bake 50 minutes.

7. Remove from oven, spread ketchup evenly over the top of the roll, and sprinkle with remaining mozzarella cheese.

8. Return to oven and bake within 10 more minutes or until cooked through and turkey reaches an internal temperature of 165°F.

9. Allow to cool and cut into six equal-sized slices. Transfer each slice to a separate airtight container and store in the refrigerator until ready to eat, up to one week.

Nutrition:
Calories: 349
Fat: 16 g
Protein: 32 g
Carbohydrates: 9 g

Mozzarella-Stuffed Turkey Meatballs

Preparation time: 15 minutes
Cooking time: 30 minutes
Servings: 6
Ingredients:

- 11/2 pounds ground turkey
- 1/2 cup minced yellow onion
- 2 cloves garlic, minced
- 1 large egg
- 1/2 cup almond meal
- 1/2 teaspoon Italian seasoning
- 1/4 cup grated Parmesan-Reggiano cheese
- 1/4 cup chopped fresh parsley
- 1 teaspoon dried basil
- 2 tablespoons chicken bone broth
- 11/2 teaspoons sea salt
- 1 teaspoon freshly ground black pepper
- 1/2 pound fresh mozzarella, cut into 18 small cubes

Directions:

1. Preheat oven to 375°F. Line a baking sheet with parchment paper. Combine all fixings, except mozzarella, in a bowl and mix with hands until incorporated.
2. Divide mixture into eighteen equal portions and form each portion into a ball; poke a hole in each meatball with your finger and stick a cheese cube inside the hole. Cover the hole by rerolling the meatball and arrange it on a prepared pan.
3. Bake within 30 minutes or until meatballs is cooked through and starting to brown. Remove from oven and allow to cool.

4. Transfer three meatballs to each of six separate airtight containers. Put in the refrigerator until ready to eat, up to one week.

Nutrition:
Calories: 336
Fat: 17 g
Protein: 32 g
Carbohydrates: 10g

Turkey Bacon Cheeseburger Meatloaf

Preparation time: 15 minutes
Cooking time: 60 minutes
Servings: 6
Ingredients:

- 6 slices no-sugar-added bacon, cooked and crumbled
- 11/2 pounds ground turkey
- 1 cup shredded Cheddar cheese
- 1 large egg
- 1 small yellow onion, peeled and diced
- 2 tablespoons coconut aminos
- 2 teaspoons granulated garlic
- 1 teaspoon dry mustard
- 1/4 teaspoon freshly ground black pepper
- 1/2 cup no-sugar-added ketchup, divided

Directions:

1. Preheat oven to 350°F. Combine all fixings, except 1/4 cup ketchup, in a medium bowl and mix with your hands until fully incorporated.
2. Transfer mixture to a 9" × 5" loaf pan and spread remaining ketchup on top. Bake 1 hour, or until internal temperature reaches 165°F. Remove from oven and allow to cool.
3. Slice into six equal portions and move each portion to a separate airtight container—store in the refrigerator for up to one week.

Nutrition:
Calories: 415
Fat: 27 g
Protein: 32 g
Carbohydrates: 9

Baked Chicken

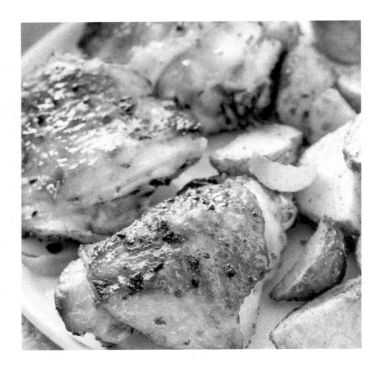

Preparation Time: 10 minutes
Cooking Time: 1 hour
Servings: 4
Ingredients:

- 3-4 pounds Chicken, cut into parts
- 3 tbsp Olive oil
- ½ tsp Thyme
- ¼ tsp Sea salt
- Ground black pepper
- ½ cup Low-sodium chicken stock

Directions:

1. Preheat the oven to 400F. Rub oil over chicken pieces. Sprinkle with salt, thyme, and pepper.
2. Place chicken in the roasting pan.
3. Bake in the oven for 30 minutes. Then lower the heat to 350F. Bake within 15 to 30 minutes more or until juice runs clear. Serve or store.

Nutrition:
Calories: 550
Fat: 19g
Carb: 0g
Protein: 91g

Orange Chicken and Broccoli Stir-Fry

Preparation Time: 10 minutes
Cooking Time: 15 minutes
Servings: 4
Ingredients:

- Olive oil – 1 Tbsp.
- Chicken breast – 1 pound, boneless and skinless, cut into strips.
- Orange juice – 1/3 cup
- Homemade soy sauce - 2 Tbsp.
- Cornstarch – 2 tsp.
- Broccoli – 2 cups, cut into small pieces.
- Snow peas – 1 cup
- Cabbage – 2 cups, shredded
- Brown rice – 2 cups, cooked
- Sesame seeds – 1 tbsp

Directions:

1. Combine the orange juice, soy sauce, and corn starch in a bowl. Set aside. Heat oil in a pan. Add chicken. Stir-fry until the chicken is golden brown on all sides, about 5 minutes.
2. Add snow peas, cabbage, broccoli, and sauce mixture. Continue to stir-fry for 8 minutes or until vegetables are tender but still crisp. Serve or store.

Nutrition:
Calories: 340
Fat: 8g
Carb: 35g
Protein: 28g

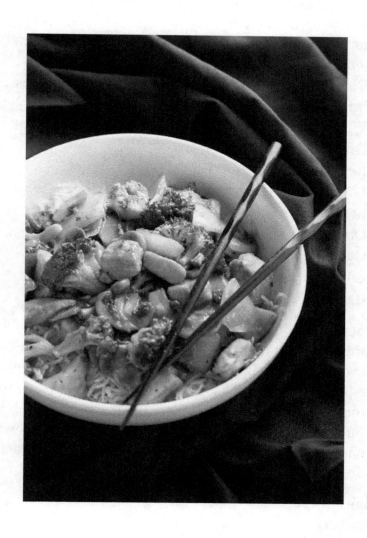

Mediterranean Lemon Chicken and Potatoes

Preparation Time: 10 minutes
Cooking Time: 30 minutes
Servings: 4
Ingredients:

- Chicken breast – 1 ½ pound, skinless and boneless, cut into 1-inch cubes
- Yukon Gold potatoes – 1 pound, cut into cubes
- Onion – 1, chopped
- Red pepper – 1, chopped
- Low-sodium vinaigrette – ½ cup
- Lemon juice – ¼ cup
- Oregano – 1 tsp.
- Garlic powder – ½ tsp.
- Chopped tomato – ½ cup
- Ground black pepper to taste

Directions:

1. Preheat oven to 400F. Except for the tomatoes, mix everything in a bowl. On 4 aluminum foils, place an equal amount of chicken and potato mixture; fold to make packets.
2. Bake at 400F for 30 minutes. Open packets. Top with chopped tomatoes. Season with black pepper to taste. Store.

Nutrition:
Calories: 320
Fat: 4g
Carb: 34g
Protein: 43g

Tandoori Chicken

Preparation Time: 10 minutes
Cooking Time: 20 minutes
Servings: 6
Ingredients:

- Nonfat yogurt – 1 cup plain
- Lemon juice – ½ cup
- Garlic – 5 cloves, crushed
- Paprika – 2 Tbsp.
- Curry powder – 1 tsp.
- Ground ginger – 1 tsp.
- Red pepper flakes – 1 tsp.
- Chicken breasts – 6, skinless and boneless, cut into 2-inch chunks.
- Wooden skewers – 6, soaked in water

Directions:

1. Preheat the oven to 400F. In a bowl, combine lemon juice, yogurt, garlic, and spices. Blend well. Divide chicken and thread onto skewers—place skewers in a baking dish.
2. Pour half of the yogurt mixture onto the chicken; cover and marinate in the refrigerator for 20 minutes. Spray a baking dish with cooking spray.
3. Place chicken skewers in the pan and coat with the remaining ½ of yogurt marinade. Bake in the oven until chicken is cooked, about 15 to 20 minutes. Serve with veggies or store.

Nutrition:
Calories: 175
Fat: 2g
Carb: 8g

Protein: 30g

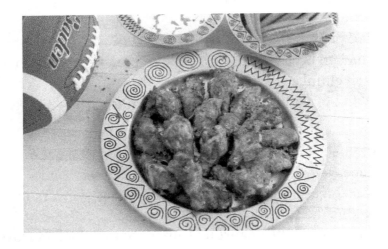

Grilled Chicken Salad

Preparation Time: 5 minutes
Cooking Time: 10 minutes
Servings: 4
Ingredients:
For the dressing:
- Red wine vinegar – ½ cup
- Garlic – 4 cloves, minced
- Extra-virgin olive oil – 1 Tbsp.
- Finely chopped red onion – 1 Tbsp.
- Finely chopped celery -1 Tbsp.
- Ground black pepper to taste

For the salad:
- Chicken breasts – 4 (4-ounce each), boneless, skinless
- Garlic – 2 cloves
- Lettuce leaves - 8 cups
- Ripe black olives – 16
- Navel oranges – 2, peeled and sliced

Directions:
1. For the dressing, combine all the dressing ingredients in a bowl and keep in the refrigerator. Heat a gas grill or broiler.
2. Lightly coat the broiler pan or grill rack with cooking spray. Position the cooking rack 4 to 6 inches from the heat source.
3. Rub the chicken breasts with garlic and discard the cloves. Broil or grill the chicken about 5 minutes per side, or until just cooked through.
4. Slice the chicken; arrange with lettuce, olives, and oranges. Drizzle with dressing and serve.

Nutrition:

Calories: 237
Fat: 9g
Carb: 12g
Protein: 27g

Ground Turkey Mini Meatloaves

Preparation Time: 10 minutes
Cooking Time: 30 minutes
Servings: 6
Ingredients:

- Lean ground turkey – 1 ½ pound
- Onion – 1, diced
- Celery – 2, diced
- Bell pepper – 1, diced
- Garlic – 4 cloves, minced
- No-salt-added tomato sauce – 1 (8-ounce) can
- Egg white – 1
- Salt-free bread crumbs – ¾ cup
- Molasses – 1 Tbsp.
- Liquid smoke – ¼ tsp.
- Freshly ground black pepper - ½ tsp.
- Salt-free ketchup – ¼ cup

Directions:
1. Preheat the oven to 375F. Spray a 6-cup muffin tin with oil and set aside. Place all ingredients except for ketchup in a bowl and mix well.
2. Fill the muffin cups with the mixture and press in firmly. Divide the ketchup between the muffin cups and spread evenly.
3. Place muffin tin on the middle rack in the oven and bake for 30 minutes. Remove, cool, and store.

Nutrition:
Calories: 251
Fat: 7g
Carb: 21g
Protein: 25g

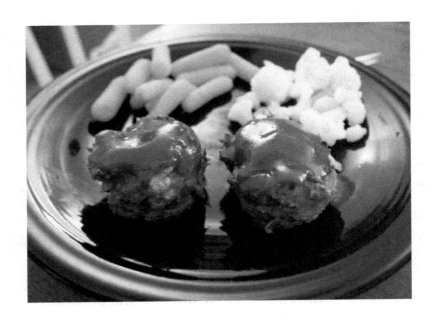

Turkey and Brown Rice Stuffed Peppers

Preparation Time: 10 minutes
Cooking Time: 35 minutes
Servings: 4
Ingredients:

- Bell peppers – 4, core and seed, leave the peppers intact
- Lean ground turkey – 1 pound
- Onion – 1, diced
- Garlic – 3 cloves, minced
- Celery – 2 stalks, diced
- Cooked brown rice – 2 cups
- No-salt-added diced tomatoes – 1 (15-ounce) can
- Salt-free tomato paste – 2 Tbsp.
- Seedless raisins – ¼ cup
- Ground cumin – 2 tsp.
- Dried oregano – 1 tsp.
- Ground cinnamon – ½ tsp.
- Ground black pepper – ½ tsp.

Directions:

1. Preheat the oven to 425F. Grease a baking pan with oil. Heat a pan over medium heat. Add onion, ground turkey, garlic, and celery and sauté for 5 minutes. Remove from heat.
2. Add the remaining ingredients and mix. Fill each pepper with ¼ of the mixture. Pressing firmly to pack.
3. Stand peppers in the prebaked baking pan, replace the pepper caps, and then cover the pan with foil. Place in the middle rack in the oven and bake for 25 to 30 minutes, or until tender. Serve.

Nutrition:
Calories: 354

Fat: 8g
Carb: 45g
Protein: 27g

Grilled Tequila Chicken with Peppers

Preparation Time: 10 minutes
Cooking Time: 30 minutes
Servings: 4
Ingredients:
- Lime juice – 1 cup
- Tequila – 1/3 cup
- Garlic – 3 cloves, chopped
- Chopped fresh cilantro – ¼ cup
- Agave nectar – 1 Tbsp.
- Ground black pepper - ½ tsp.
- Cumin – 1 tsp.
- Ground coriander – ½ tsp.
- Boneless, skinless chicken breasts – 4
- Olive oil – 2 tsp.
- Green bell pepper – 1, diced
- Red bell pepper – 1, diced
- Onion – 1, diced
- Nonfat sour cream – ½ cup

Directions:
1. In a bowl, add the lime juice, tequila garlic, cilantro, agave nectar, black pepper, cumin, and coriander and mix well.
2. Add the chicken breasts and coat well. Cover and marinate them for at least 6 hours (in the refrigerator).
3. Heat the grill—Cook the chicken for 10 to 15 minutes per side, or no longer pink. Meanwhile, heat the oil in a pan.
4. Add the pepper and onion—Stir-fry for 5 minutes. Remove from heat. Remove chicken from the grill; serve with veggies and sour cream.

Nutrition:
Calories: 259
Fat: 3g
Carb: 18g
Protein: 28g

Orange-Rosemary Roasted Chicken

Preparation Time: 10 minutes
Cooking Time: 45 minutes
Servings: 6
Ingredients:

- Chicken breast halves – 3, skinless, bone-in, each 8 ounces
- Chicken legs with thigh pieces – 3, skinless, bone-in, each 8 ounces
- Garlic cloves – 2, minced
- Extra-virgin olive oil – 1 ½ tsp.
- Fresh rosemary – 3 tsp.
- Ground black pepper – 1/8 tsp.
- Orange juice – ½ cup

Directions:

1. Preheat oven at 450F. Grease a baking pan with cooking spray. Rub chicken with garlic, then with oil. Sprinkle with pepper and rosemary. Put the chicken pieces in the baking dish, then pour the orange juice.
2. Cover and bake for 30 minutes, then flip the chicken with tongs and cook 10 to 15 minutes more or until browned. Baste the chicken with the pan juice from time to time. Serve chicken with pan juice.

Nutrition:
Calories 204
Fat: 8g
Carb: 2g
Protein: 31g

Honey Crusted Chicken

Preparation Time: 10 minutes
Cooking Time: 25 minutes
Servings: 2
Ingredients:

- Saltine crackers – 8, (2-inch square each) crushed
- Paprika – 1 tsp.
- Chicken breasts – 2, boneless, skinless (4-ounce each)
- Honey – 4 tsp.
- Cooking spray to grease a baking sheet

Directions:

1. Preheat the oven to 375F. In a bowl, mix crushed crackers and paprika. Mix well. In another bowl, add honey and chicken. Coat well.
2. Add to the cracker mixture and coat well. Put the chicken on your prepared baking sheet. Bake for 20 to 25 minutes. Serve.

Nutrition:
Calories: 219
Fat: 3g
Carb: 21g
Protein: 27g

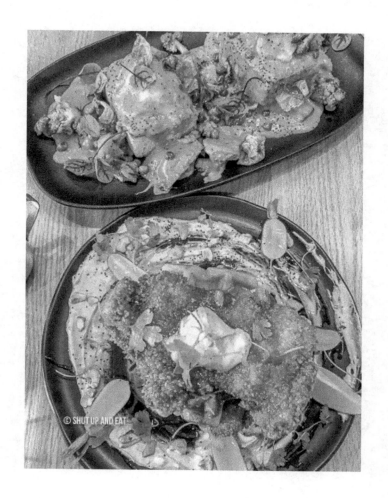

CPSIA information can be obtained
at www.ICGtesting.com
Printed in the USA
BVHW040036200421
605310BV00009B/774